Selfish Mom Project

A 60-Day Guide to Being Selfish & Finding Yourself

Rachael Tapper

www.SelfishMomProject.com

Formatting by Daniel J. Mawhinney

www.40DayPublishing.com

Cover design by Jonna Feavel Thames

www.40DayGraphics.com

Printed in the United States of America

Contents

To my precious reader:

As I write this intro to you on my phone, I have currently locked myself in the bathroom while one dog is staring at me, one set of hands is trying to unlock the door knob, and another set of precious hands is reaching under the door for me. My almost preteen daughter is texting me to please let her have TikTok on her phone…"where am I again"? My phone is at three-percent battery and I'm currently begging/praying to God to not let my phone die and to freely give me the words that all you sweet mommas need to hear.

If you're anything like me you are exhausted. You're tired. You're wondering how in the heck are you supposed to become a selfish mom and find yourself when you just had your first shower in four days.

I promise you miracles do happen and prayers are answered every day and for some reason this sixty-day guidebook is calling to you.

My wish for you as you go through the next sixty days is that you understand just how important you are. That you find your oxygen mask and fully secure it before you touch anyone else's. That you understand the magnitude of the quote:

"I am the only person who can give my children a happy mother."

November 1, 2017, I decided to take control of taking care of myself first. I began the first ever Selfish Mom Project.

I'd love to tell you the idea came about in a professional fashion, but really it was a couple weeks earlier after a few bottles of wine with friends, and me knee-deep in postpartum depression after having our third child, Max.

I was so stuck in suck when the slurred words, "I just need to be selfish every once in a while. Why doesn't anyone understand that? You know what, I'm going to do a Selfish Mom Project and be selfish every day for sixty days." The next morning, with a hangover that I'm most definitely not proud of, my husband decided to remind me of my Selfish Mom Project...and was I really going to do it? Not one to stand down to a challenge I assured him (and my kids!) I would most definitely be doing this project. I was starting November 1st the following week.

Knowing that I had to hold myself accountable in some way, I decided to post about it on my social media accounts. I know myself (and maybe you're the same)—I needed the extra accountability to stick to the entire sixty days. For four years I had shown my accountability through a network marketing company I was part of and it had always done its job to keep me accountable publicly.

I felt this project for myself was no different. I posted my recent struggles with going from two to three kids, the overwhelm I was feeling along with the crippling anxiety, and the fact that I was having some really dark days. Even worse, that I was really good at hiding it and keeping it all together, but I knew I was struggling with some serious postpartum depression and I needed help.

The outreach from my social media post was amazing. At a point where I felt so alone in my journey as a mother, I found myself in a sea of women who could relate, were ready to cheer me on, and follow my journey. Over the course of the next sixty days I received hundreds of emails and messages on social media. Some cheering me on and others of moms who were desperately struggling with the same issues of losing yourself in the midst of motherhood that I was.

Two years later, I sit here and I write this manual as a kick-starter for any mom out there struggling with finding her place in motherhood. I take that back. I write this for any mom out there that frankly just wants to find a place for herself in HER actual LIFE.

THIS IS YOUR LIFE, MOMMAS. You will see it several times throughout this guidebook:

YOU ARE THE ONLY PERSON WHO CAN GIVE YOUR KIDS A HAPPY MOM.

You're going to have to stand up, be a little selfish, take the time, and DO the work to find your best self.

I hope you use this sixty-day journey to fully come into your truth. Find your worth. Notice all the moments of happiness and progress, even the small ones, because there will be days where it's hard to see.

I hope this guide helps you not just take care of you but find you.

That is my hope, you exhausted momma.

Remember, you are loved. You are special. You are a great mom even if you don't know how to cut a sandwich the right way and can't read their precious tiny little minds. And most importantly remember that you are truly worthy of greatness, success, and the ability to love and take care of yourself.

Xoxo you wonderful momma,

Rachael Tapper

Four Selfish Mom Love Languages

When I started my own journey on the Selfish Mom Project I thought my days would consist of mani/pedis, facials, and ladies who lunch. I quickly realized that not only would my bank account not allow for sixty days of this but in reality that's not what I actually needed. I needed to learn to love myself in a new way.

I found in the first three days that there were FOUR love languages that I needed to personally hit each day to feel my best: SOCIAL, EMOTIONAL, PHYSICAL, & SPIRITUAL. There's no particular order; they are all equally important. For me and most of the clients I work with, these love languages need to be fulfilled each day.

Social:

Like Elizabeth Taylor would say, "Get up, get dressed, and put on some lipstick." Okay, you really don't have to do all of those things, but you need to make sure you're making a social effort to society each day. I struggle with what I call a hermit or hibernation phase a couple times a year and have to force myself to leave the house. Sometimes it's because I'm in total creation/work mode or sometimes it's because I genuinely don't want to make the effort to see people. The latter is when I know I've been slacking in my social SMP love languages.

There is such a culture of having a 'mom tribe' or a pack of friends. I've found that to not only be hard but to also be incredibly intimidating. Instead, the idea here is to encourage you to step outside your comfort zone every once in a while...leave the house, join a club, take off the yoga pants (yes, I know they are cozy but they too deserve a break)...and make an effort to be social with someone that is over forty-two inches tall. Your brain deserves to work in a different, new, more challenging way, by having conversations with adults.

As amazing as I think mom groups are, I also find that I need a group of people to surround myself with that have absolutely nothing to do with my children. YOU ARE NOT OBLIGATED TO BE BFFS with your kid's friend's parents. I feel so much better that I just wrote that because being a new mom, or any kind of mom for that matter, there can be a lot of pressure to 'fit in' with the other moms on the playground. Make sure you're making an attempt to be social with a variety of groups. You'll thank yourself later when the last thing you feel like discussing is sleeping schedules and colors of poop. One day your kids are going to leave the nest and you need to be able to have conversations that don't revolve around your kids.

Emotional:

Filling the emotional cup is one of my favorites, yet also one of the hardest. It's so easy to do that you can actually forget to do it. In the next couple of sections we will talk more about establishing a mindset routine for yourself, and this is exactly where I think the emotional aspect of the SMP love languages should fit in.

The emotional love language is meant to be therapeutic. Most of my days are spent kissing boo-boos, listening to preteen drama, or watching one if not all three of my kiddos have an absolute meltdown. Sometimes I look at them and have just a twinge of jealousy that they are able to melt down and it's completely expected of them, almost okay, for them to do it. We are constantly calming our children, asking them to use their words, but busy moms tell me they don't have time to feel, they must move too quickly on to the next phase of the day. There is no space or time in their day to 'release' their emotions. What I noticed while working with my clients and myself was how easy it is for us to hide our emotions. At thirty-five years old, there are plenty of days I'm tested into whether or not I'm able to fully express my emotions. This is why the emotional love language is so important and should not be overlooked. Even after kissing all the boo-boos, my emotions deserve the ability to release and be heard even if it's just in my journal. Just because I'm a mom doesn't mean I have to put on a brave face all the time. I'm allowed to cry, stomp my feet, and feel disappointment. It's a natural state of life, right? I've found kicking my feet and screaming are not the most mature route, so instead I choose to find gratitude and do journal therapy daily. I have designed this guide to be a space for you to record what I call the Gratitude Five daily and will have journal prompts throughout. I highly recommend finding a journal that suits you and your needs. Taking ten minutes at some point in your day to simply journal how you're feeling will instantly release built-up emotions.

Physical:

I feel like this is a little bit more self-explanatory than some of the other SMP love languages, but mommas, we gotta move our bodies. This is not me telling you to strive to be a size anything. This is me simply telling you to show your body gratitude. I don't know a lot about cars, but I do know (from learning the hard way) that when a light comes on you need to get that checked out! Our bodies are designed for movement. Whether it's fifteen minutes a day or you check into an Orangetheory class five days a week, it makes no difference to me. Start small and maybe work to something greater or maybe be completely content with those precious ten minutes of movement you give yourself each day.

Spiritual:

The spiritual love language is all about connecting to a higher power than yourself. As moms, society puts pressure on us that we must be able to do it all. First of all, it's not even possible, and secondly, I've found that the best guidance always comes from a higher power than myself. For me personally that means hitting my knees daily and praying to God for guidance. After my prayer I sit in meditation for five to ten minutes...nothing crazy, just something to give the big guy upstairs a moment to guide my heart and mind in the direction I need to be going.

The SMP spiritual love language has been the most impactful on my life to date. Some days it will be hard to find that moment of quiet that you need, but I know that truly this is one love language that I cannot miss a day of. I've had so many of my clients say quiet time is hard to come by and they have a hard time settling their minds down because they keep thinking of all the things they need to be doing instead of sitting and asking for guidance. This is totally normal, and after two years of taking a moment each day, I still find there are days I struggle really hard with this. Don't let it discourage you; just show up daily for the practice.

How to use this guidebook

Unlike motherhood, this guidebook is not meant to be complicated. Think of it as a daily check-in with yourself. For the next sixty days, you will be checking in with yourself in this planner using the Four Selfish Mom Love Languages.

This isn't about implementing everything at once. If your life is anything like mine, it's not going to allow it. You can start slow or dive right in. The choice is yours. Though the guidebook is suggested for sixty days of growth by finding daily selfish time and yourself, don't ever feel the pressure, the obligation, or, especially, the guilt if you miss a day. Come back when you're ready.

The guidebook is laid out like a planner to give you a daily opportunity to check in with yourself. How fulfilled do you feel? Were you able to hit those Four Selfish Mom Love Languages? I'll break up the days throughout the guidebook with check-ins, my own stories of struggle and motherhood, and journal prompts to get you moving to the next level of growth.

You will notice that each page includes a space for you to write out your Gratitude Five list, check in with your four love languages, write a special affirmation or mantra for yourself, and a space for your to-do list. I have only left a space for three things on your to-do list. Yes, just three. Motherhood is overwhelming already; let's not make it harder. Adding a to-do list three pages deep doesn't help out in any way. By only giving three spaces for you, I want you to release the sense of overwhelm and keep things simple. Super simple. On the next page of the book, you will find a brain-dump page. This is a page for your master to-do list. The goal is each day or week pick three things to accomplish and not feel overwhelmed by a massive list. If you are in a particularly busy season of motherhood, I highly recommend taking a moment each Sunday night to plan out your up-coming week. See what lies ahead and where you can insert yourself in your days.

Remember, motherhood might be complicated but taking care of yourself doesn't have to be.

Feel free to go to the resources section of this book at any time for additional ideas and guidance, or you can always reach out to me at www.selfishmomproject.com.

Create Your Master To-Do List

You'll notice I only gave space for three things to be added to your to-do list each day. This sixty-day journey should be simple and mostly focused on you. I don't want you loading it up with volunteering and being at your family's beck and call. I want you to find space in your already crazy day to take care of yourself on the inside and out. In order to do that, I truly believe you need to limit the tasks you take on and limit your to-do list to a maximum of three tasks a day. Scribble up this page with all the tasks you need to get done and make this your master list that you are able to pull from daily. Think of this as a place to completely dump your brain out.

My recommendation would be to mark this page, as you will come back to it almost daily.

1.

2.

3.

4.

5.

6.

7.

8.

9.

10.

11.

12.

13.

14.

15.

16.

17.

18.

19.

20.

21.

22.

23.

24.

25.

26.

27.

28.

29.

30.

31.

32.

33.

34.

35.

36.

37.

38.

39.

40.

41.

42.

43.

44.

45.

46.

47.

48.

49.

50.

51.

52.

53.

54.

55.

56.

57.

58.

59.

60.

SELFISH MOM PROJECT

DAILY CHECK IN

GRATITUDE FIVE

1.

2.

3.

4.

5.

AFFIRMATION OR MANTRA FOR TODAY

DAILY TO DO LIST

- [ ]
- [ ]
- [ ]

- [ ] MOVED MY BODY
- [ ] MY SPIRITUAL PRACTICE
- [ ] CONNECTED WITH OTHERS
- [ ] TEN MINUTES OF JOURNALING

SELFISH MOM PROJECT

DAILY CHECK IN

GRATITUDE FIVE

1.

2.

3.

4.

5.

AFFIRMATION OR MANTRA FOR TODAY

DAILY TO DO LIST

- [ ]
- [ ]
- [ ]

- [ ] MOVED MY BODY
- [ ] MY SPIRITUAL PRACTICE
- [ ] CONNECTED WITH OTHERS
- [ ] TEN MINUTES OF JOURNALING

SELFISH MOM PROJECT

DAILY CHECK IN

GRATITUDE FIVE

1.
2.
3.
4.
5.

AFFIRMATION OR MANTRA FOR TODAY

DAILY TO DO LIST

- [ ]
- [ ]
- [ ]

- [ ] MOVED MY BODY
- [ ] MY SPIRITUAL PRACTICE
- [ ] CONNECTED WITH OTHERS
- [ ] TEN MINUTES OF JOURNALING

SELFISH MOM PROJECT

DAILY CHECK IN

GRATITUDE FIVE

1.

2.

3.

4.

5.

AFFIRMATION OR MANTRA FOR TODAY

DAILY TO DO LIST

- [ ]
- [ ]
- [ ]

- [ ] MOVED MY BODY
- [ ] MY SPIRITUAL PRACTICE
- [ ] CONNECTED WITH OTHERS
- [ ] TEN MINUTES OF JOURNALING

SELFISH MOM PROJECT

DAILY CHECK IN

GRATITUDE FIVE

1.
2.
3.
4.
5.

AFFIRMATION OR MANTRA FOR TODAY

DAILY TO DO LIST

- [ ]
- [ ]
- [ ]

- [ ] MOVED MY BODY
- [ ] MY SPIRITUAL PRACTICE
- [ ] CONNECTED WITH OTHERS
- [ ] TEN MINUTES OF JOURNALING

SELFISH MOM PROJECT

DAILY CHECK IN

GRATITUDE FIVE

1.

2.

3.

4.

5.

AFFIRMATION OR MANTRA FOR TODAY

DAILY TO DO LIST

- [ ]
- [ ]
- [ ]

- [ ] MOVED MY BODY
- [ ] MY SPIRITUAL PRACTICE
- [ ] CONNECTED WITH OTHERS
- [ ] TEN MINUTES OF JOURNALING

SELFISH MOM PROJECT

DAILY CHECK IN

GRATITUDE FIVE

1.
2.
3.
4.
5.

AFFIRMATION OR MANTRA FOR TODAY

DAILY TO DO LIST

- [ ]
- [ ]
- [ ]

- [ ] MOVED MY BODY
- [ ] MY SPIRITUAL PRACTICE
- [ ] CONNECTED WITH OTHERS
- [ ] TEN MINUTES OF JOURNALING

Establishing a Mindset Routine

You are the only person who can give your kids a happy mom.

I told you this affirmation would come up everywhere, right? This is truly one of my favorite affirmations. Every day at 6:42 am a little ping goes off on my phone reminding me of this special and amazing quote. Stop imagining me jumping out of bed being perky and giving my kids these warm "Get up sleepy head" vibes. It's not like that every day, but this affirmation does help start my day off in a better way.

There is nothing worse than waking up in the best mood only to have a kid lose their minds, or a grumpy spouse, turning your awesome mood into a rotten one. This can happen anytime throughout the day, actually.

My middle child used to determine my mood on the daily...and let's just be clear, he rarely wakes up in a good mood (not a morning person at all) and (whoa) after school he can be a handful depending on if he got a sticker or not. No matter what I did, some days I just couldn't make it right, and it would end up ruining my day too.

I made the decision that no one, especially if you can't tie your shoes by yourself, was allowed to determine my mood for the day.

I realized early in my first Selfish Mom Project I was going to have to establish some daily rituals and boundaries that would help mold me to how I wanted to feel daily. Rituals that were strong enough to take me through the day and that I could continuously call on throughout the day. The mind is tricky but also something you can shape with habits you form daily. I learned in this process that protecting my mindset and energy was precious—not always easy, but it was something I had to do daily in order to take care of myself and be a happier mom and partner.

1. Pray - It doesn't get more free or cost-effective than this, folks. Prayer is free, and in return it's freeing for your soul. I start every single day by praying to the big guy upstairs for patience, peace, safety, and sanity. Don't just save prayer for once a day. He's not going anywhere...why not reach out throughout the day when you're feeling yourself slip.

2. Gratitude - I've written in a gratitude journal for six years now and it's one of my favorite parts of the day. It takes five minutes, and it reminds me of even the smallest things that I have to be grateful for. During the bad seasons of life it's forgotten we are actually living extraordinary lives. How many times have you truly been

grateful for clean water?! That's not an option for a lot of people in the world. Finding gratitude is a precious gift.
Of course, there will be difficult days or rough seasons, but I bet if you dig really deep you'll find it.

3. Journaling - Or I like to call it FREE THERAPY. I'm not knocking therapy at all; been there and done that for years. Journal therapy, as I call it, has become just as effective (and it's free) as actually going. It's releasing any predisposition as to what may come out on paper and just allowing the thoughts to roll into the pen and transfer to paper. This can be so meditative after a solid prayer. I've talked myself out of lots of bad decisions, negative mindsets, and tough situations through journal therapy.

4. Daily Dance Party - Almost daily we have a dance party at the Tapper house. I grew up in the early years of my life at a radio station and music has always been a place for me to just let loose. It can also help me release almost any emotion I'm holding in. It can help me cry, smile, get pumped up, and get some rest. Ever have a horrible day and your favorite song comes on the radio and it totally makes your day? Imagine stopping for just a second every morning and doing just that. We like to jam out on the way to school, and I love watching my kiddos jump out of the car with a little pep in their step due to jamming out to something that raised their vibration and mood just a little bit. Music is a spirit lifter...even if you're in a major funk.

5. Meditation - I wish I could gift this to the world and that everyone truly understood the importance of meditation.

It's easy, free, and will completely change your life. The opportunity to find absolute stillness and silence in the present moment is so hard when you are a mom, but I promise if you can find this one little moment in your day it will change your life for the better. Meditation is proven to reduce stress and anxiety. Dedicating just five minutes a day to clearing all thoughts and lists out of your head and sitting with yourself will teach you a lot and earn you some patience points as well.

Journal Prompt:

HOW IS YOUR MINDSET IN THE MORNING, AND HOW DOES IT CHANGE THROUGHOUT THE DAY? TAKE FIVE TO TEN MINUTES AND WRITE ABOUT HOW YOUR MOODS CHANGE THROUGHOUT THE DAY, WHAT TRIGGERS THEM, AND HOW THESE TOOLS CAN BE CONTINUOUSLY USED TO CHANGE ANY NEGATIVE MINDSET THAT MIGHT COME IN THROUGHOUT THE DAY.

SELFISH MOM PROJECT

DAILY CHECK IN

GRATITUDE FIVE

1.
2.
3.
4.
5.

AFFIRMATION OR MANTRA FOR TODAY

DAILY TO DO LIST

- [ ]
- [ ]
- [ ]

- [ ] MOVED MY BODY
- [ ] MY SPIRITUAL PRACTICE
- [ ] CONNECTED WITH OTHERS
- [ ] TEN MINUTES OF JOURNALING

SELFISH MOM PROJECT

DAILY CHECK IN

GRATITUDE FIVE

1.

2.

3.

4.

5.

AFFIRMATION OR MANTRA FOR TODAY

DAILY TO DO LIST

- [ ]
- [ ]
- [ ]

- [ ] MOVED MY BODY
- [ ] MY SPIRITUAL PRACTICE
- [ ] CONNECTED WITH OTHERS
- [ ] TEN MINUTES OF JOURNALING

SELFISH MOM PROJECT

DAILY CHECK IN

GRATITUDE FIVE

1.
2.
3.
4.
5.

AFFIRMATION OR MANTRA FOR TODAY

DAILY TO DO LIST

- [ ]
- [ ]
- [ ]

- [ ] MOVED MY BODY
- [ ] MY SPIRITUAL PRACTICE
- [ ] CONNECTED WITH OTHERS
- [ ] TEN MINUTES OF JOURNALING

SELFISH MOM PROJECT

DAILY CHECK IN

GRATITUDE FIVE

1.

2.

3.

4.

5.

AFFIRMATION OR MANTRA FOR TODAY

DAILY TO DO LIST

- [ ]
- [ ]
- [ ]

- [ ] MOVED MY BODY
- [ ] MY SPIRITUAL PRACTICE
- [ ] CONNECTED WITH OTHERS
- [ ] TEN MINUTES OF JOURNALING

SELFISH MOM PROJECT

DAILY CHECK IN

GRATITUDE FIVE

1.

2.

3.

4.

5.

AFFIRMATION OR MANTRA FOR TODAY

DAILY TO DO LIST

- [ ]
- [ ]
- [ ]

- [ ] MOVED MY BODY
- [ ] MY SPIRITUAL PRACTICE
- [ ] CONNECTED WITH OTHERS
- [ ] TEN MINUTES OF JOURNALING

SELFISH MOM PROJECT

DAILY CHECK IN

GRATITUDE FIVE

1.

2.

3.

4.

5.

AFFIRMATION OR MANTRA FOR TODAY

DAILY TO DO LIST

- [ ]
- [ ]
- [ ]

- [ ] MOVED MY BODY
- [ ] MY SPIRITUAL PRACTICE
- [ ] CONNECTED WITH OTHERS
- [ ] TEN MINUTES OF JOURNALING

SELFISH MOM PROJECT

DAILY CHECK IN

GRATITUDE FIVE

1.

2.

3.

4.

5.

AFFIRMATION OR MANTRA FOR TODAY

DAILY TO DO LIST

- [ ]
- [ ]
- [ ]

- [ ] MOVED MY BODY
- [ ] MY SPIRITUAL PRACTICE
- [ ] CONNECTED WITH OTHERS
- [ ] TEN MINUTES OF JOURNALING

You deserve the opportunity to take care of yourself.

Congrats, momma...you've made it through the first couple weeks! Are you finding it easy or hard to get through all your love languages daily? Today I'm here to remind you that you deserve these sixty days.

Every single momma deserves the opportunity to take care of herself. She deserves all her Selfish Mom Love Languages to be met daily. The same as our kids expect food, water, milk, hugs, and a warm home filled with love...YOU, MOMMA, deserve the opportunity to take care of yourself.

I'm currently writing this as I heat up three different meals (leftover night) and my husband is on a fishing trip because I want you to understand that there are going to be days, months, maybe years where making yourself and your wellbeing a priority are going to be hard. It will feel impossible. Like it can't be done. Like you have no support. Like this is just life and this is just the way it's going to be...someday my time will come.

No, right NOW is your time. There will never be a right time. There will never be a perfect moment or season of motherhood. You're gonna have to work with what God gave you, and that's this exact moment.

It might be easy and it might not be. You're gonna have to call in the troops. That might be your mom tribe or that might be having a really hard conversation with your partner and family, or it might be starting from scratch and finding a support system that will really work for you and with you.

I like to call this theory the Empty Cup Theory.

Not long after I had our third baby, and days before I started the first Selfish Mom Project, I remember cooking dinner while wearing a baby and helping with homework. I sat down to eat dinner and someone asked me for something. Got up to get it, sat back down. Someone asked for something else, I got up and got it...the routine continued until I finally sat down to eat cold food, nursing while I ate, his sweet head covered in crumbs I had dropped. The theory hit me straight in the head when someone at the table asked if I could get them more water. I realized I hadn't even gotten myself a drink. I brought in a pitcher of water and an extra glass and slammed it down on the table. Everyone looked up at me, shocked. I explained my empty cup theory to my family. This big pitcher of water was Mommy. Starting off full, but since everyone needed some attention, time, or just something from me, I had to pour myself out into their glass. See Jay's cup getting full, Sophia's cup getting full, Daddy needs me too, and now we have Max, who is little and needs a lot of my time, as I poured water into the glass I slammed down till it overflowed onto the kitchen table. Everyone looked at me as I pointed to the pitcher of water—empty. Empty was how I felt, and I told them that. I needed help from all of them. At first I felt bad that it was a lot of pressure to put on my children. At eight and four, were they really ready to take on more responsibility? Does this make me a bad mom because I wasn't able to be at their beck and call? No, this made me a better mom because I needed the time each day to fill my cup. I think of my sweet children and what this process I have brought into our lives has taught them. I hope mostly my daughter sees a mother that not only loves and takes care of her but also loves and takes care of herself.

If you get one thing from this journey over the next sixty days, I hope it's that you understand that you are worthy of taking care of yourself...FIRST. Your cup should always feel full.

Journal Prompt:

WHERE ARE YOU FINDING IN YOUR WEEK YOU ARE STRUGGLING TO COMPLETE THE DAILY SELFISH MOM LOVE LANGUAGES? TAKE FIVE TO TEN MINUTES ON WHY YOU ARE WORTHY ENOUGH TO COMPLETE THE ENTIRE SIXTY DAYS OF THIS CHALLENGE.

SELFISH MOM PROJECT

DAILY CHECK IN

GRATITUDE FIVE

1.

2.

3.

4.

5.

AFFIRMATION OR MANTRA FOR TODAY

DAILY TO DO LIST

- [ ]
- [ ]
- [ ]

- [ ] MOVED MY BODY
- [ ] MY SPIRITUAL PRACTICE
- [ ] CONNECTED WITH OTHERS
- [ ] TEN MINUTES OF JOURNALING

SELFISH MOM PROJECT

DAILY CHECK IN

GRATITUDE FIVE

1.
2.
3.
4.
5.

AFFIRMATION OR MANTRA FOR TODAY

DAILY TO DO LIST

- [ ]
- [ ]
- [ ]

- [ ] MOVED MY BODY
- [ ] MY SPIRITUAL PRACTICE
- [ ] CONNECTED WITH OTHERS
- [ ] TEN MINUTES OF JOURNALING

SELFISH MOM PROJECT

DAILY CHECK IN

GRATITUDE FIVE

1.
2.
3.
4.
5.

DAILY TO DO LIST

- [ ]
- [ ]
- [ ]

- [ ] MOVED MY BODY
- [ ] MY SPIRITUAL PRACTICE
- [ ] CONNECTED WITH OTHERS
- [ ] TEN MINUTES OF JOURNALING

AFFIRMATION OR MANTRA FOR TODAY

SELFISH MOM PROJECT

DAILY CHECK IN

GRATITUDE FIVE

1.

2.

3.

4.

5.

AFFIRMATION OR MANTRA FOR TODAY

DAILY TO DO LIST

- [ ]
- [ ]
- [ ]

- [ ] MOVED MY BODY
- [ ] MY SPIRITUAL PRACTICE
- [ ] CONNECTED WITH OTHERS
- [ ] TEN MINUTES OF JOURNALING

SELFISH MOM PROJECT

DAILY CHECK IN

GRATITUDE FIVE

1.

2.

3.

4.

5.

AFFIRMATION OR MANTRA FOR TODAY

DAILY TO DO LIST

- [ ]
- [ ]
- [ ]

- [ ] MOVED MY BODY
- [ ] MY SPIRITUAL PRACTICE
- [ ] CONNECTED WITH OTHERS
- [ ] TEN MINUTES OF JOURNALING

SELFISH MOM PROJECT

DAILY CHECK IN

GRATITUDE FIVE

1.

2.

3.

4.

5.

AFFIRMATION OR MANTRA FOR TODAY

DAILY TO DO LIST

- [ ]
- [ ]
- [ ]

- [ ] MOVED MY BODY
- [ ] MY SPIRITUAL PRACTICE
- [ ] CONNECTED WITH OTHERS
- [ ] TEN MINUTES OF JOURNALING

SELFISH MOM PROJECT

DAILY CHECK IN

GRATITUDE FIVE

1.

2.

3.

4.

5.

AFFIRMATION OR MANTRA FOR TODAY

DAILY TO DO LIST

- [ ]
- [ ]
- [ ]

- [ ] MOVED MY BODY
- [ ] MY SPIRITUAL PRACTICE
- [ ] CONNECTED WITH OTHERS
- [ ] TEN MINUTES OF JOURNALING

Release All the Guilt

Mom Guilt. It's like regular guilt, but instead it completely consumes us and makes it damn near impossible to enjoy any part of being a mom, let alone our life outside of motherhood (which you should be starting to establish at this point).

Y'all, if there is one section in this guidebook that you read twice, please, for the love of all things good in the world, let it be this one. We as a society of moms have got to release the guilt we place on ourselves and each other.

I suffered with a lot of postpartum depression after each of my kids, and I think it's because I always knew I wanted to do something besides being a mother. I felt bad for feeling that way, for wanting of course to be a mom but to also have something else in my life, whether that was a passion or a career. Each of my children got to have me home with them their first year of life, and though I'm so blessed I was able to do that, those years were hard. I felt guilty for wanting a life outside of them. I felt guilty that I was not able to financially contribute in the way I wanted to our family. Double guilt. Even worse, because I was so hung up on all the guilt, I started resenting everyone around me and placing blame on them and then back on myself. It's a vicious cycle, and so many moms out there are living it.

Mom guilt is bad. Literally one of the worst feelings in the world. As a society of mothers, we are letting it steal our precious moments of motherhood away from us. Not only just our motherhood, WE ARE ALLOWING it to steal the joy out of our life in general!

Did you know you can book a hotel room by yourself and stay in it, sleep in it, wake up the next day, come home, and still be an awesome mom?

Did you know that booking a sitter so that you and your partner can go out for a night will not only make you a good mom, BUT will probably also give you an opportunity to reconnect with that sexy person you fell so in love with. Nothing is hotter that having sex above a whisper and easy conversation that's not interrupted by someone saying "mom" every five seconds.

Did you know that booking a girls trip, getting a mani/pedi, missing a school function/party, or (God forbid) making your kid eat a lunch where the sandwich is not cut into the shape of a cute animal will still make you a good mother?

Did you know that having a career or job or passion that you love and are excited to go to everyday STILL makes you a good mother?

I have a theory about mom guilt. Mom guilt just shows how much we love our kids. We love them so much that we are willing to pull out all the Pinterest stops and put ourselves last so that we don't feel guilty when they are without something or without us. The theory proves how much we love our children, but it doesn't prove how much we love and care for ourselves and our spiritual, mental, emotional, physical, and social wellbeing. I want my kids to know I love them more than anything, but I also want them to know how to love and take care of themselves by being an example for them.

Release all the mom guilt, knowing that being a little selfish and taking time for you actually gives you the opportunity to recharge your circuit and come back, being your best self. Sometimes we are so laser-focused on the mom guilt that we don't see the places or moments we are nailing this motherhood thing. You are an amazing mom, no matter how many times you go to work, on a vacation with your spouse, miss a school function, or leave to go get a manicure.

Here is your permission to release alllllll the guilt.

Journal Prompt:

WHERE DOES MOM GUILT COME INTO YOUR LIFE? SPEND FIVE TO TEN MINUTES WRITING ON WHERE YOU FIND YOURSELF STRUGGLING WITH MOM GUILT AND HOW IT SHOWS UP IN YOUR LIFE. FOLLOW UP WITH WRITING THE WAYS YOU SHOW UP AS AN AWESOME MOM.

SELFISH MOM PROJECT

DAILY CHECK IN

GRATITUDE FIVE

1.

2.

3.

4.

5.

AFFIRMATION OR MANTRA FOR TODAY

DAILY TO DO LIST

- [ ]
- [ ]
- [ ]

- [ ] MOVED MY BODY
- [ ] MY SPIRITUAL PRACTICE
- [ ] CONNECTED WITH OTHERS
- [ ] TEN MINUTES OF JOURNALING

SELFISH MOM PROJECT

DAILY CHECK IN

GRATITUDE FIVE

1.

2.

3.

4.

5.

DAILY TO DO LIST

- [ ]
- [ ]
- [ ]

AFFIRMATION OR MANTRA FOR TODAY

- [ ] MOVED MY BODY
- [ ] MY SPIRITUAL PRACTICE
- [ ] CONNECTED WITH OTHERS
- [ ] TEN MINUTES OF JOURNALING

SELFISH MOM PROJECT

DAILY CHECK IN

GRATITUDE FIVE

1.

2.

3.

4.

5.

AFFIRMATION OR MANTRA FOR TODAY

DAILY TO DO LIST

- [ ]
- [ ]
- [ ]

- [ ] MOVED MY BODY
- [ ] MY SPIRITUAL PRACTICE
- [ ] CONNECTED WITH OTHERS
- [ ] TEN MINUTES OF JOURNALING

SELFISH MOM PROJECT

DAILY CHECK IN

GRATITUDE FIVE

1.
2.
3.
4.
5.

DAILY TO DO LIST

- [ ]
- [ ]
- [ ]

- [ ] MOVED MY BODY
- [ ] MY SPIRITUAL PRACTICE
- [ ] CONNECTED WITH OTHERS
- [ ] TEN MINUTES OF JOURNALING

AFFIRMATION OR MANTRA FOR TODAY

SELFISH MOM PROJECT

DAILY CHECK IN

GRATITUDE FIVE

1.

2.

3.

4.

5.

AFFIRMATION OR MANTRA FOR TODAY

DAILY TO DO LIST

- [ ]
- [ ]
- [ ]

- [ ] MOVED MY BODY
- [ ] MY SPIRITUAL PRACTICE
- [ ] CONNECTED WITH OTHERS
- [ ] TEN MINUTES OF JOURNALING

SELFISH MOM PROJECT

DAILY CHECK IN

GRATITUDE FIVE

1.
2.
3.
4.
5.

AFFIRMATION OR MANTRA FOR TODAY

DAILY TO DO LIST

- [ ]
- [ ]
- [ ]

- [ ] MOVED MY BODY
- [ ] MY SPIRITUAL PRACTICE
- [ ] CONNECTED WITH OTHERS
- [ ] TEN MINUTES OF JOURNALING

SELFISH MOM PROJECT

DAILY CHECK IN

GRATITUDE FIVE

1.
2.
3.
4.
5.

DAILY TO DO LIST

- [ ]
- [ ]
- [ ]

- [ ] MOVED MY BODY
- [ ] MY SPIRITUAL PRACTICE
- [ ] CONNECTED WITH OTHERS
- [ ] TEN MINUTES OF JOURNALING

AFFIRMATION OR MANTRA FOR TODAY

The Art of Saying No

I'm currently in a season of saying no, and I love it!

At first it wasn't easy (insert mom guilt), but I noticed that the more I started saying it, the less I was asked to do things that, frankly, I didn't enjoy.

Don't get me wrong. I want to be there for every moment for my kids, but not when it produces an unhappy and overwhelmed momma. This is exactly why there are only three things on your daily to-do list.

I used to think that I wanted to volunteer for each thing at all their schools. I wanted to go to every moms' night out, party, and event. Some would say I suffer from FOMO (fear of missing out) ...or we can just go back to the mom guilt section here.

I realized that sometimes showing up for these things weren't actually serving me in a positive manner...it was making me miserable. In turn, making me super resentful to my kids and husband for making me feel like I had to say yes to all the things, places, parties, and demands.

It's a struggle at first to say no.

I made the conscious decision a while back to Marie Kondo my decision-making skills—if something did not bring me joy, I was out...not going to do it. Even if that meant saying no to volunteering at my kid's school. My kids will physically live a pretty good life and survive if I'm not able to make it to every single thing they do. The world will still spin when I cancel all plans because I see the state of my family and realize that soccer practice is not a good choice. I promise.

I found yoga when I was five months pregnant with our third child. I fell in love, and yoga was a great way for me to get several of my Selfish Mom Love Languages met. In fall of 2018, I made the decision to put myself into a two hundred-hour yoga teacher training program. That meant that for Two hundred hours in eight months, I was going to be away from my family. Two weekends every month, I left my kids and husband to indulge in my passion and love for yoga. Five to six classes a week, I was carrying my children off to sit in childcare while I took a class. Numerous times, my ego and mom guilt popped into my head, making me feel bad for putting all this parenting responsibility on my husband, missing sports games, school functions, and asking on my mom tribe to pick up my slack. It was eight months of saying no to a lot of things and people so that I could say yes to myself. What I learned was that my husband was pretty darn good at juggling three kids solo. I had an amazing support system, and my kids were thriving, proud of me and not resentful. I took those eight months to heal some past wounds, and yoga teacher training ended up being one of the best things I ever did. Though it will not always be easy, sometime we must say no to others in order to say yes to ourselves.

Journal Prompt:

WHAT NO LONGER BRINGS YOU JOY THAT YOU IN THE PAST WOULD HAVE SAID YES TO? CAN YOU SAY NO TO IT? FIND FIVE TO TEN MINUTES TODAY TO LOOK AT THE WEEK AHEAD AND ALL THE THINGS YOU HAVE SAID YES TO IN THE FUTURE. WRITE ABOUT WHETHER THEY TRULY BRING YOU JOY AND THE STEPS YOU CAN TAKE TO START SAYING NO TO THEM AND YES TO YOURSELF.

SELFISH MOM PROJECT

DAILY CHECK IN

GRATITUDE FIVE

1.

2.

3.

4.

5.

AFFIRMATION OR MANTRA FOR TODAY

DAILY TO DO LIST

- [ ]
- [ ]
- [ ]

- [ ] MOVED MY BODY
- [ ] MY SPIRITUAL PRACTICE
- [ ] CONNECTED WITH OTHERS
- [ ] TEN MINUTES OF JOURNALING

SELFISH MOM PROJECT

DAILY CHECK IN

GRATITUDE FIVE

1.

2.

3.

4.

5.

AFFIRMATION OR MANTRA FOR TODAY

DAILY TO DO LIST

- [ ]
- [ ]
- [ ]

- [ ] MOVED MY BODY
- [ ] MY SPIRITUAL PRACTICE
- [ ] CONNECTED WITH OTHERS
- [ ] TEN MINUTES OF JOURNALING

SELFISH MOM PROJECT

DAILY CHECK IN

GRATITUDE FIVE

1.

2.

3.

4.

5.

AFFIRMATION OR MANTRA FOR TODAY

DAILY TO DO LIST

- [ ]
- [ ]
- [ ]

- [ ] MOVED MY BODY
- [ ] MY SPIRITUAL PRACTICE
- [ ] CONNECTED WITH OTHERS
- [ ] TEN MINUTES OF JOURNALING

SELFISH MOM PROJECT

DAILY CHECK IN

GRATITUDE FIVE

1.

2.

3.

4.

5.

AFFIRMATION OR MANTRA FOR TODAY

DAILY TO DO LIST

- [ ]
- [ ]
- [ ]

- [ ] MOVED MY BODY
- [ ] MY SPIRITUAL PRACTICE
- [ ] CONNECTED WITH OTHERS
- [ ] TEN MINUTES OF JOURNALING

SELFISH MOM PROJECT

DAILY CHECK IN

GRATITUDE FIVE

1.

2.

3.

4.

5.

AFFIRMATION OR MANTRA FOR TODAY

DAILY TO DO LIST

- [ ]
- [ ]
- [ ]

- [ ] MOVED MY BODY
- [ ] MY SPIRITUAL PRACTICE
- [ ] CONNECTED WITH OTHERS
- [ ] TEN MINUTES OF JOURNALING

SELFISH MOM PROJECT

DAILY CHECK IN

GRATITUDE FIVE

1.

2.

3.

4.

5.

AFFIRMATION OR MANTRA FOR TODAY

DAILY TO DO LIST

- [ ]
- [ ]
- [ ]

- [ ] MOVED MY BODY
- [ ] MY SPIRITUAL PRACTICE
- [ ] CONNECTED WITH OTHERS
- [ ] TEN MINUTES OF JOURNALING

SELFISH MOM PROJECT

DAILY CHECK IN

GRATITUDE FIVE

1.

2.

3.

4.

5.

AFFIRMATION OR MANTRA FOR TODAY

DAILY TO DO LIST

- [ ]
- [ ]
- [ ]

- [ ] MOVED MY BODY
- [ ] MY SPIRITUAL PRACTICE
- [ ] CONNECTED WITH OTHERS
- [ ] TEN MINUTES OF JOURNALING

Pinterest is a B

I saw a meme the other day on Facebook that said, "There are two types of moms in the world...the Pinterest mom and the Amazon Prime mom." I certainly hate that we as a society have categorized an entire population of mothers into two categories. If we are being honest though, in this season of my life I'm a proud Amazon Prime mom, and 100% okay with that. Let's all express some gratitude to the inventor of Amazon that we don't have to put on a bra to go buy toilet paper anymore. You don't have to put yourself in either of these categories; maybe you're a mixture of both or neither! The point is that we have to be okay with whatever 'box' we decide to put ourselves in and own it.

When I was a new mom, I loved Martha Stewart. I would put Sophia to bed, pour a glass of wine, and literally devour every single page of the magazine. Often the same magazine several times that month. In our crappy, dingy, dirty, DC apartment, I would dream up all the things I would do one day when I had a gorgeous house and unlimited funds to decorate. Pinterest then was merely a site you had to get on a waiting list for, reserved for cool bloggers, and soon I found myself checking my email multiple times a day trying to see if finally made the cut. The magical day came, and I became sucked into the site like a Cheerio in a vacuum cleaner.

I was hooked. I spent hours a day pinning different boards, dreaming of my perfect body, my one-day dream home, all the crafts I was going to do with my perfectly dressed little humans, and the magical meal that would pop right off my Pinterest board on to the plates of my family who gobbled it up just like the title said they would.

None of this happened. I'll inform you right now, I was so busy pinning away I missed all the opportunities I had to work out and get my perfect body with two kids. The crafts became overwhelming, and did you know there is no Pinterest fairy that comes to help you scrub off the gallons of glitter and glue a four-year-old can pour out in five seconds? My dinners didn't only not pop out of the screen, but often set off the smoke detector in our apartment building because...well, a lot of reasons, but I like to think every oven is different. My dream home was nowhere in sight, and when it did finally come in to play, I was so overwhelmed with the idea of decorating due to Pinterest boards that it literally sat barren for years. Five, to be exact, as I have just now started figuring out the style I like through magazines and a designer rather than relying on different Pinterest boards.

Pinterest became a sense of overwhelm for me. I felt like a failure every time something just didn't come out, taste well, or look pretty. I started going hard-core on the comparison game and realized that Pinterest was stealing my joy...not only out of being a mother but in being myself!

Before all the moms that identify with being a Pinterest mom out there start bashing my book, I want to say I applaud you. One mom in particular jumps to mind when I think Pinterest mom. My cousin Cassie. Cassie has five kids (and at the time I'm writing this) is pregnant with her sixth. I love when she posts pictures of anything that has a theme. She is truly a creative genius! You can tell her kids love it; they enjoy it...there's a thorough process that goes behind it all. Most importantly, you can see that SHE LOVES DOING IT. She is not apologetic about it. She owns it and loves it. She also talks a lot unapologetically about the difficulty of being a mom and how much she relies on God's grace to get her through the different phases of motherhood. I love how she owns the (amazing) motherhood phase she is in.

There is NOTHING wrong with being either mom—or some other type of mom, for that matter. It gets wrong when it doesn't serve you in a positive way. For me in my season of life, Amazon Prime serves me in a positive way, and Pinterest serves me negatively. That wasn't always the case, but today it is. It makes my heart skip a beat and happy knowing that I can order something to solve the problem and it will be here in a two-hour delivery time window with no added shipping fee. Maybe for you it is making something beautiful and being that Pinterest mom—whatever it is, it shouldn't stress you out or put you in the comparison mode. You should love every minute of it.

If you're like me and maybe feel the pressures that society puts on us as moms to make extravagant valentine boxes and that's just really not your thing...do yourself a favor and delete the app from your phone. I felt no shame whatsoever when I bought my kids a premade box from Target—and guess what? I'm still able to cook a mediocre dinner after deleting the app. Do I still get on Pinterest? Yes, but it's with a mindset that it's fun and I don't have to play the comparison game...I certainly don't have to feel obligated to do any of it.

Journal Prompt:

HAVE YOU EVER FELT THE PRESSURE FROM OTHER MOTHERS TO DO THINGS A CERTAIN WAY? WHAT KIND OF MOM DO YOU THINK YOU ARE? DO YOU OWN IT, OR DO YOU FIND YOURSELF LIVING IN THE COMPARISON GAME?

SELFISH MOM PROJECT

DAILY CHECK IN

GRATITUDE FIVE

1.
2.
3.
4.
5.

AFFIRMATION OR MANTRA FOR TODAY

DAILY TO DO LIST

- [ ]
- [ ]
- [ ]

- [ ] MOVED MY BODY
- [ ] MY SPIRITUAL PRACTICE
- [ ] CONNECTED WITH OTHERS
- [ ] TEN MINUTES OF JOURNALING

SELFISH MOM PROJECT

DAILY CHECK IN

GRATITUDE FIVE

1.

2.

3.

4.

5.

AFFIRMATION OR MANTRA FOR TODAY

DAILY TO DO LIST

- [ ]
- [ ]
- [ ]

- [ ] MOVED MY BODY
- [ ] MY SPIRITUAL PRACTICE
- [ ] CONNECTED WITH OTHERS
- [ ] TEN MINUTES OF JOURNALING

SELFISH MOM PROJECT

DAILY CHECK IN

GRATITUDE FIVE

1.

2.

3.

4.

5.

AFFIRMATION OR MANTRA FOR TODAY

DAILY TO DO LIST

- [ ]
- [ ]
- [ ]

- [ ] MOVED MY BODY
- [ ] MY SPIRITUAL PRACTICE
- [ ] CONNECTED WITH OTHERS
- [ ] TEN MINUTES OF JOURNALING

SELFISH MOM PROJECT

DAILY CHECK IN

GRATITUDE FIVE

1.

2.

3.

4.

5.

AFFIRMATION OR MANTRA FOR TODAY

DAILY TO DO LIST

- [ ]
- [ ]
- [ ]

- [ ] MOVED MY BODY
- [ ] MY SPIRITUAL PRACTICE
- [ ] CONNECTED WITH OTHERS
- [ ] TEN MINUTES OF JOURNALING

SELFISH MOM PROJECT

DAILY CHECK IN

GRATITUDE FIVE

1.

2.

3.

4.

5.

AFFIRMATION OR MANTRA FOR TODAY

DAILY TO DO LIST

- [ ]
- [ ]
- [ ]

- [ ] MOVED MY BODY
- [ ] MY SPIRITUAL PRACTICE
- [ ] CONNECTED WITH OTHERS
- [ ] TEN MINUTES OF JOURNALING

SELFISH MOM PROJECT

DAILY CHECK IN

GRATITUDE FIVE

1.

2.

3.

4.

5.

DAILY TO DO LIST

- [ ]
- [ ]
- [ ]

- [ ] MOVED MY BODY
- [ ] MY SPIRITUAL PRACTICE
- [ ] CONNECTED WITH OTHERS
- [ ] TEN MINUTES OF JOURNALING

AFFIRMATION OR MANTRA FOR TODAY

SELFISH MOM PROJECT

DAILY CHECK IN

GRATITUDE FIVE

1.
2.
3.
4.
5.

AFFIRMATION OR MANTRA FOR TODAY

DAILY TO DO LIST

- [ ]
- [ ]
- [ ]

- [ ] MOVED MY BODY
- [ ] MY SPIRITUAL PRACTICE
- [ ] CONNECTED WITH OTHERS
- [ ] TEN MINUTES OF JOURNALING

Finding Humor in Motherhood

On the last day of 2018, I said a small prayer.

I asked God that no matter what happened in our life this year that we always trust in his guidance and that he always found a way to make us laugh.

I read a quote (I'm not sure who it's from) that simply stated, "Once you start laughing, you start healing." I knew in 2019 I needed to do some physical and mental healing. I had started slacking in my love languages, and I could witness it in my marriage and in the eyes of my children. I needed more laughing and healing and less fretting the small stuff.

As mothers, we go through about a million emotions in one day. It's easy to laugh when our kids are doing something silly, and it's hard to find a giggle when you're stuck in suck and having a rough parenting day/week/month/year, but it's essential to healing and growing.

Laughter and humor are how we heal, and healing is how we grow—grow into a better version of ourselves. The Four Selfish Mom Project Love Languages were designed to help you grow. They might not be easy to complete daily, but they are essential, and I'm adding laughter as a bonus love language because I think it's that important.

It's not always going to be super obvious at first to find the humor, even in the super stressful situations. I have found that they are almost like a test. Some days you're going to have to look really hard to find laughter.

Our daughter has a very hard time adjusting to different altitudes and gets super carsick. As a family of five, we drive to pretty much all our destinations (it's cheaper) and she absolutely hates it. Two days after this prayer to God about finding humor in all aspects of life, I found my first test. Forty-five minutes into our ten-hour drive from Colorado to Texas, Sophia started saying she didn't feel good. We slightly ignored her (she's a little dramatic). I took video of the snow falling, commenting the temperature was so much colder as we descended the mountain. Less than an hour into our drive, Sophia started to tell us to pull over...and instead she turned to baby Max in the car seat next to her and, exorcist style, threw up all over him. I will never forget that small moment of pure silence before all three kids started screaming and Dino and I started scrambling on where to pull over (literally, we were driving on a mountain). We drove for several miles before we finally found a bank parking lot to pull over and change two of our three kids in. I probably looked like a crazy person changing my poor sick daughter in thirteen-degree weather in a bank parking lot, laughing hysterically. Legit crazy. The thing is, that situation could have gone one of two ways. I could have freaked out and lost my cool on everyone and made a (very) long car trip with three kids seem even more miserable, or I could have taken it as an 'oh well' moment and just laughed. Sophia threw up the rest of the trip, and no, I did not laugh the rest of those times. Of course I felt horrible for her, but knowing that I was able to find humor in a really crappy (and smelly) situation made what ended up being a fifteen-hour car ride a little more bearable.

I keep two funny videos of my kids in my 'favorites' section of my phone and come back to them often when myself or someone in the family is having a funky or bad day. It can be hard to find the humor but always keep a look out for an opportunity to laugh. I hope you always choose to grow through laughter.

Journal Prompt:

WRITE ABOUT A FUNNY PARENTING MOMENT! REMEMBERING IS THE FIRST STEP! WHERE HAVE YOU MISSED A MOMENT OF HUMOR? HOW COULD YOU OPEN YOURSELF UP TO MORE LAUGHTER AND GROWING AND LESS STRESS AND OVERWHELM?

SELFISH MOM PROJECT

DAILY CHECK IN

GRATITUDE FIVE

1.

2.

3.

4.

5.

AFFIRMATION OR MANTRA FOR TODAY

DAILY TO DO LIST

- [ ]
- [ ]
- [ ]

- [ ] MOVED MY BODY
- [ ] MY SPIRITUAL PRACTICE
- [ ] CONNECTED WITH OTHERS
- [ ] TEN MINUTES OF JOURNALING

SELFISH MOM PROJECT

DAILY CHECK IN

GRATITUDE FIVE

1.

2.

3.

4.

5.

AFFIRMATION OR MANTRA FOR TODAY

DAILY TO DO LIST

- [ ]
- [ ]
- [ ]

- [ ] MOVED MY BODY
- [ ] MY SPIRITUAL PRACTICE
- [ ] CONNECTED WITH OTHERS
- [ ] TEN MINUTES OF JOURNALING

SELFISH MOM PROJECT

DAILY CHECK IN

GRATITUDE FIVE	DAILY TO DO LIST
1.	☐
2.	☐
3.	☐
4.	
5.	

AFFIRMATION OR MANTRA FOR TODAY

- ☐ MOVED MY BODY
- ☐ MY SPIRITUAL PRACTICE
- ☐ CONNECTED WITH OTHERS
- ☐ TEN MINUTES OF JOURNALING

SELFISH MOM PROJECT

DAILY CHECK IN

GRATITUDE FIVE

1.

2.

3.

4.

5.

AFFIRMATION OR MANTRA FOR TODAY

DAILY TO DO LIST

- [ ]
- [ ]
- [ ]

- [ ] MOVED MY BODY
- [ ] MY SPIRITUAL PRACTICE
- [ ] CONNECTED WITH OTHERS
- [ ] TEN MINUTES OF JOURNALING

SELFISH MOM PROJECT

DAILY CHECK IN

GRATITUDE FIVE

1.
2.
3.
4.
5.

AFFIRMATION OR MANTRA FOR TODAY

DAILY TO DO LIST

- [ ]
- [ ]
- [ ]

- [ ] MOVED MY BODY
- [ ] MY SPIRITUAL PRACTICE
- [ ] CONNECTED WITH OTHERS
- [ ] TEN MINUTES OF JOURNALING

SELFISH MOM PROJECT

DAILY CHECK IN

GRATITUDE FIVE

1.

2.

3.

4.

5.

AFFIRMATION OR MANTRA FOR TODAY

DAILY TO DO LIST

- [ ]
- [ ]
- [ ]

- [ ] MOVED MY BODY
- [ ] MY SPIRITUAL PRACTICE
- [ ] CONNECTED WITH OTHERS
- [ ] TEN MINUTES OF JOURNALING

SELFISH MOM PROJECT

DAILY CHECK IN

GRATITUDE FIVE

1.

2.

3.

4.

5.

AFFIRMATION OR MANTRA FOR TODAY

DAILY TO DO LIST

- [ ]
- [ ]
- [ ]

- [ ] MOVED MY BODY
- [ ] MY SPIRITUAL PRACTICE
- [ ] CONNECTED WITH OTHERS
- [ ] TEN MINUTES OF JOURNALING

It's Okay to Not Always Like This

I've been pretty open about my parenting journey on social media. I've used it a little as a diary because I love the concept of Facebook memories each year reminding me about some really precious moments but also some really hard ones. The hard ones are a reminder of how much I have grown or maybe where I still need to do the work.

I started to look back on some of the moments I have shared. Especially taking a closer look at some of those not so great moments I have shared. It never fails someone out there always comments on the post, " You're going to miss this one day!"

Ugh. This is always so frustrating to me when people say this. I know I am going to miss this, but maybe right now in this moment I'm not liking this. I think it is really okay to say that too a few times. It's okay for me to practice getting my emotions as a mother out, even if they're not necessarily positive. Being a mom and motherhood is not always positive! Right now I'm watching my child throwing himself on the floor again for the umpteenth time today and me carrying him out of Whole Foods like a surfboard—I don't like this right now. I don't need to hear I'm going to miss this...I need someone to hug me and tell me it's okay to not like being a mom today. I need someone to tell me I'm doing a good job even when it doesn't feel like it and I'm not loving it.

There's too much pressure on moms to enjoy every single second of motherhood. Yes, it is a wonderful joy and a precious opportunity to be a mother. I am forever grateful for the opportunity and ability to have three wonderful kids that God blessed me with. But let's get this straight. It's hard too. Like the hardest job out there. I'm never going to be that mom to lie to social media with perfectly filtered pictures and sweet stories of my kids and their outfits and make people believe that I love every single second of this motherhood gig every single day.

I don't. That doesn't mean I love my children any less, or that you do either. What it means is, instead of commenting that one day I'll miss whatever it is that today, I'm just having a bad parenting day. Tell me tomorrow will be better, give me a hug, and pour me a big glass of wine.

And yes, we probably will miss all this, even the really hard days, one day, but until then I support you in your decision to not like today or not like being a mom today. I know you love your children. I'm offering a big cheers and a virtual hug and holding a special place for you on the hard days when you are not feeling this mothering gig.

Journal Prompt:

REFLECT BACK ON A DAY THAT YOU JUST DIDN'T LIKE AS A MOTHER.

SELFISH MOM PROJECT

DAILY CHECK IN

GRATITUDE FIVE

1.
2.
3.
4.
5.

AFFIRMATION OR MANTRA FOR TODAY

DAILY TO DO LIST

- [ ]
- [ ]
- [ ]

- [ ] MOVED MY BODY
- [ ] MY SPIRITUAL PRACTICE
- [ ] CONNECTED WITH OTHERS
- [ ] TEN MINUTES OF JOURNALING

SELFISH MOM PROJECT

DAILY CHECK IN

GRATITUDE FIVE

1.

2.

3.

4.

5.

AFFIRMATION OR MANTRA FOR TODAY

DAILY TO DO LIST

- [ ]
- [ ]
- [ ]

- [ ] MOVED MY BODY
- [ ] MY SPIRITUAL PRACTICE
- [ ] CONNECTED WITH OTHERS
- [ ] TEN MINUTES OF JOURNALING

SELFISH MOM PROJECT

DAILY CHECK IN

GRATITUDE FIVE

1.

2.

3.

4.

5.

AFFIRMATION OR MANTRA FOR TODAY

DAILY TO DO LIST

- [ ]
- [ ]
- [ ]

- [ ] MOVED MY BODY
- [ ] MY SPIRITUAL PRACTICE
- [ ] CONNECTED WITH OTHERS
- [ ] TEN MINUTES OF JOURNALING

SELFISH MOM PROJECT

DAILY CHECK IN

GRATITUDE FIVE

1.

2.

3.

4.

5.

AFFIRMATION OR MANTRA FOR TODAY

DAILY TO DO LIST

- [ ]
- [ ]
- [ ]

- [ ] MOVED MY BODY
- [ ] MY SPIRITUAL PRACTICE
- [ ] CONNECTED WITH OTHERS
- [ ] TEN MINUTES OF JOURNALING

SELFISH MOM PROJECT

DAILY CHECK IN

GRATITUDE FIVE

1.

2.

3.

4.

5.

AFFIRMATION OR MANTRA FOR TODAY

DAILY TO DO LIST

- [ ]
- [ ]
- [ ]

- [ ] MOVED MY BODY
- [ ] MY SPIRITUAL PRACTICE
- [ ] CONNECTED WITH OTHERS
- [ ] TEN MINUTES OF JOURNALING

SELFISH MOM PROJECT

DAILY CHECK IN

GRATITUDE FIVE

1.
2.
3.
4.
5.

AFFIRMATION OR MANTRA FOR TODAY

DAILY TO DO LIST

- [ ]
- [ ]
- [ ]

- [ ] MOVED MY BODY
- [ ] MY SPIRITUAL PRACTICE
- [ ] CONNECTED WITH OTHERS
- [ ] TEN MINUTES OF JOURNALING

SELFISH MOM PROJECT

DAILY CHECK IN

GRATITUDE FIVE

1.

2.

3.

4.

5.

AFFIRMATION OR MANTRA FOR TODAY

DAILY TO DO LIST

- [ ]
- [ ]
- [ ]

- [ ] MOVED MY BODY
- [ ] MY SPIRITUAL PRACTICE
- [ ] CONNECTED WITH OTHERS
- [ ] TEN MINUTES OF JOURNALING

Selfishly Advocating for Your Own Health

As we near the end of this journey together, I am assuming you have started making progress daily in putting yourself first or at least on your to-do list.

When our kids are sick, we drop everything to care for them. We rush to the store, buying popsicles and medicine; we compromise our own immunity for the extra snuggles they need and change sheets covered in Lord knows what in the middle of the night. We selflessly give everything to make our babies feel better.

But there is no rest for the momma who's feeling under the weather or hitting a wall of exhaustion that no amount of sleep can take care of. There's no rest for the momma who can list a million symptoms or who knowingly knows somethings just seems 'off'.

As mothers, we are built on a strong intuition of our children's health. We know when it's serious or maybe when they just need some extra attention. But what's our intuition on our own health? Are we checking in the way we should by doing yearly checkups, or are we brushing it off as just the stress of motherhood?

I'm not talking about mental health here, though mental health awareness should always be at the top of our list...I'm talking about our physical health. This entire process, we should have been working on our mental health, but we can't forget to check in with our physical health every once in a while.

Seven years ago, I began a journey into my physical health. I had a two-and-a-half-year old child living in bustling DC while my husband and I worked eighty-plus-hour workweeks for our recently acquired new restaurant. I was busy, I was exhausted, I found my twenty-four-year-old body feeling crippled every morning when I woke. And then I found a little round lump in my throat. Insert freak-out moment and me booking the next available doctor's appointment. You know what the biggest problem was? I didn't even have a primary doctor because, well, I'm the mom and it never occurred to me that my health or finding a doctor was something I needed to do. Thankfully, I did find that doctor, and the cause for that tiny lump after tons of tests was never determined to be anything to worry about.

Fast-forward through the years where different unknown aliments came and went that no doctor could explain and made me feel crazier by the day. Through the years I found myself excusing most of these symptoms as, "I'm a mom of course I'm exhausted (or insert all other aliments I was dealing with." In seven years, I have struggled with severe hair loss, low libido, excessive weight gain (and weight loss), extreme fatigue, anxiety, and depression. By the age of thirty-five, I'd had four mammograms (none covered by insurance) due to unknown lumps, and was told I just have lumpy breasts. I've had extreme crippling joint pain, migraines, multiple swollen lymph nodes, food intolerance, and generally, just feeling of suck. I went to lots of doctors. All kinds of doctors. I was poked and prodded. I was tested for many autoimmune diseases, extreme fatigue disorder, thyroid issues, MS, and even Lupus! Every single blood test, scan, and mammogram came back telling me I was a poster mom for health. Then why did I constantly feel like crap and couldn't make it through a day without a nap?

I remember at one point asking my husband, "What's wrong with me? I feel like my body is just shutting down."

Mommas, just like you are an advocate for your children's health and wellbeing, you are also an advocate for your own health. If something doesn't feel right, keep searching...don't accept that it's just motherhood. Your health is just as important.

I'm thankful for a friend that encouraged me to keep digging. I came across a website talking about Breast Implant Illness. Having breast implants for over fifteen years, I never thought something that was so common in today's society could be the result of any of the symptoms I was having. But as I looked through the list of symptoms, I realized I was checking almost every single box. I immediately booked with a plastic surgeon to discuss the options for getting them out ASAP.

September 18th, 2019, I made the decision to evict the saline implants that had made their home in my body for the last fifteen years. Within days, my health and energy level had improved drastically. So much so, my six-year-old told me my skin was beautiful. Of course, not all of my symptoms have completely gone away...detox takes time. I can 100% assure you that, had I not been an advocate for my own health, I'd still be struggling with my health and not being the best possible mom I could be.

This isn't about having or not having breast implants or how they are bad, this is about you being SELFISH enough to put your health first. If something doesn't feel right, don't allow others to dismiss how you feel, you're not crazy, you know your body.

We are given one body. Just one. Listen to it. Be selfish with it and know that YOU are the only person who can truly advocate for your health. Your children need you happy, but they also need you healthy.

Journal Prompt:

MAKE A LIST OF PAST DUE APPOINTMENTS FOR YOUR HEALTH THAT YOU HAVE POSSIBLY BEEN NEGLECTING. NOW EITHER CALL OR FIND A PROVIDER THAT YOU CAN MAKE APPOINTMENTS WITH.

SELFISH MOM PROJECT

DAILY CHECK IN

GRATITUDE FIVE

1.

2.

3.

4.

5.

AFFIRMATION OR MANTRA FOR TODAY

DAILY TO DO LIST

- [ ]
- [ ]
- [ ]

- [ ] MOVED MY BODY
- [ ] MY SPIRITUAL PRACTICE
- [ ] CONNECTED WITH OTHERS
- [ ] TEN MINUTES OF JOURNALING

SELFISH MOM PROJECT

DAILY CHECK IN

GRATITUDE FIVE

1.
2.
3.
4.
5.

AFFIRMATION OR MANTRA FOR TODAY

DAILY TO DO LIST

- [ ]
- [ ]
- [ ]

- [ ] MOVED MY BODY
- [ ] MY SPIRITUAL PRACTICE
- [ ] CONNECTED WITH OTHERS
- [ ] TEN MINUTES OF JOURNALING

SELFISH MOM PROJECT

DAILY CHECK IN

GRATITUDE FIVE

1.
2.
3.
4.
5.

AFFIRMATION OR MANTRA FOR TODAY

DAILY TO DO LIST

- [ ]
- [ ]
- [ ]

- [ ] MOVED MY BODY
- [ ] MY SPIRITUAL PRACTICE
- [ ] CONNECTED WITH OTHERS
- [ ] TEN MINUTES OF JOURNALING

SELFISH MOM PROJECT

DAILY CHECK IN

GRATITUDE FIVE

1.

2.

3.

4.

5.

AFFIRMATION OR MANTRA FOR TODAY

DAILY TO DO LIST

- [ ]
- [ ]
- [ ]

- [ ] MOVED MY BODY
- [ ] MY SPIRITUAL PRACTICE
- [ ] CONNECTED WITH OTHERS
- [ ] TEN MINUTES OF JOURNALING

SELFISH MOM PROJECT

DAILY CHECK IN

GRATITUDE FIVE

1.

2.

3.

4.

5.

AFFIRMATION OR MANTRA FOR TODAY

DAILY TO DO LIST

- [ ]
- [ ]
- [ ]

- [ ] MOVED MY BODY
- [ ] MY SPIRITUAL PRACTICE
- [ ] CONNECTED WITH OTHERS
- [ ] TEN MINUTES OF JOURNALING

SELFISH MOM PROJECT

DAILY CHECK IN

GRATITUDE FIVE

1.

2.

3.

4.

5.

AFFIRMATION OR MANTRA FOR TODAY

DAILY TO DO LIST

- [ ]
- [ ]
- [ ]

- [ ] MOVED MY BODY
- [ ] MY SPIRITUAL PRACTICE
- [ ] CONNECTED WITH OTHERS
- [ ] TEN MINUTES OF JOURNALING

SELFISH MOM PROJECT

DAILY CHECK IN

GRATITUDE FIVE

1.

2.

3.

4.

5.

AFFIRMATION OR MANTRA FOR TODAY

DAILY TO DO LIST

- [ ]
- [ ]
- [ ]

- [ ] MOVED MY BODY
- [ ] MY SPIRITUAL PRACTICE
- [ ] CONNECTED WITH OTHERS
- [ ] TEN MINUTES OF JOURNALING

This is it. The end.

Hopefully you have made it this far. Hopefully you were able to laugh, cry, relate to this book, and maybe even start opening up an honest conversation with yourself, your family, and others around you.

Hopefully you were able to get started on the journey to finding yourself outside of motherhood.

See being a selfish mom isn't about all the manis and pedis that are about to be on your agenda. Those are nice, and if you can, please try and fit them in—they will make you feel good—but this level of selfish, it's so much more than that. It's about your mental and physical health and the opportunity to put yourself back in your life.

It's about knowing that you are more than one role. Not just a mom.

That you are worthy of whatever you want out of life, whether that is to be a mom or maybe something more. You shouldn't have to apologize for wanting to be both or either. My mother always said, "I've done my job right if you want to leave the nest one day."

This process and journey is about continually growing and aspiring to be better but also feeling grateful and content with the season you're in. Even when it's a hard one.

Being a selfish mom is knowing that it's okay to take care of yourself first. Whether is physically, mentally, socially, or spiritually, it doesn't matter. You deserve to explore all those options.

I'll say it one last time...

YOU ARE THE ONLY PERSON WHO CAN GIVE YOUR KIDS A HAPPY MOM.

Only YOU! I don't care if you have thirty minutes or thirty seconds a day to focus on yourself. You deserve it! If you still don't believe it this far in, think of your children. Your children deserve to have a mom who is happy. Life is going to throw you one sucky season of parenting after the next. It's up to you to fight back and say I matter. When the mean girls come, when you're still not sleeping through the night (Lord, what is wrong with this kid!), when they leave for their first date, or go to college...whatever the season you're in, it's not a punishment, it's an opportunity to learn a new lesson about yourself and grow more. Lean into the tough days with prayer and asking for guidance. Find time daily for your Selfish Mom Love Languages. Find a community that lifts you up and supports you and loves you in three-day old yoga pants.

Always remember that you have to make yourself a priority so that you can be the best version of yourself for those snotty little people that throw tantrums in the grocery store. On the days that are long and you feel so lonely, gross, and unloved, oh, you sweet mom, I love you. Each morning I pray for the tribe of moms who will someday read this book. I pray they know their worth, how important they truly are, and that they aspire to be great because God has given us the most important job of all.

We are mothers.

Resources

Affirmations for Moms

I am exactly the mom my children need.

I am enough.

I am worthy of taking care of myself in any and all capacities I need.

I do not have to be perfect to be a good parent.

I am a good mom.

I am capable of amazing things.

I have the power to make any day a great day.

My kids do not need a perfect mom.

I speak kind words to myself.

I am calm even in the midst of chaos.

I call on a higher power to guide me daily.

I am not "just" a mom.

I am thankful for this day.

My children are safe and happy because of me.

What I accomplished today was enough, and I am satisfied that I did my best.

I am releasing stress and worry from my mind and replacing it with peace.

This too shall pass.

I fully embrace today.

I will find humor and laugh today.

My role as a mother is worth millions.

I am leaving a legacy of love for my children.

I love myself.

I will take care of myself.

It's okay to ask for help.

I participate in what I can and feel good about releasing the rest.

I have the permission to change.

Today I choose to live in gratitude.

I am in charge of being calm, no matter how my child behaves.

I will let go of how I think today is supposed to go and accept how it imperfectly happens.

I see the beauty in chaos.

Rachael Tapper

Everything I need is already inside me.

Yesterday's failures do not determine my today.

I cannot pour from an empty cup; today I choose to take time to fill mine.

I say no to the things that do not serve me.

I am special and do not feel the need to compare myself to other moms.

Playlists

This is my personal playlist that gets me pumped up about life.

"Girl on Fire" by Alicia Keys

"I am Here" by P!nk

"Just the Way You Are" by Bruno Mars

"Thunder" by Imagine Dragons (pretty much anything by them we jam out to!)

"Don't Stop Believin'" by Journey

"Firework" by Katy Perry

"F**king Perfect" by P!nk (they have an edited version)

"You Say" by Lauren Daigle

"Shake it Off" by Taylor Swift

"This is Why We Can't Have Nice Things" by Taylor Swift

"Confident" by Demi Lovato

"Chandelier" by Sia

"Titanium" by David Guetta (feat. Sia)

"You're Worthy of it All" by Shane & Shane

"Talk" by Daya

Anything Tom Petty because we are obsessed

"Run the World (Girls)" by Beyonce

Rachael Tapper

"We Are the Champions" by Queen

"Going Bad" by Mill Creek (feat. Drake)

"The Middle" by Zedd, Maren Morris

"God's Plan" by Drake

"BOOM" by Tiesto

"With Lifted Hands" by Ryan Stevenson

Greatest Showman Soundtrack

"Anything" by Will T Willy Waves

50 Ways to be Selfish

Book yourself a night in a hotel

Snuggle up with a good book

Meditate

Journal

Book a girls' trip

Girls'-night-out dinner

Send your partner off with the kids for a trip and stay home

Do a brain dump

Take a day off work

Go to bed early

Make a bucket list

Watch a chick flick

Spend an hour on your hobby

Take a walk

Have sex

Write a list of compliments to yourself

Buy yourself flowers

Work out or take a class (yoga is my fave)

Bake your favorite treat

Order dessert

Make a date night each week for a month!

Mani/Pedi

Book a facial

Book a massage

Declutter a space in your home or office

Do something that makes you laugh

Take a bath with sea salts and candles

Go on a retreat

Turn your phone off for the day

Have a virtual coffee date with a friend not close by

Write yourself a love letter

Book yourself a wellness checkup

Take yourself out to lunch alone

Find a new hobby or something you have always wanted to do

Take a nap

Sleep in

Stay in your pajamas all day

Get dressed up and hit the town

Cook a fancy meal

Spend time in gratitude

Walk in the grass barefoot

Have a picnic

Go to a concert

Put money aside just to spend on you

Do something you've always wanted to do

Make a vision board

Get your hair done

Take a moment to stop and be present and mindful

Say no to something that is not bringing you joy

Release any guilt or negative feelings you may be having

About the Author:

Rachael Tapper is a self-proclaimed selfish mom to three kids and married for a million years to the love of her life; they reside in Dallas, Texas. The founder of the Selfish Mom Project, Rachael has made it her life's mission to encourage moms to selfishly love themselves and remind them to secure their own oxygen mask first. She loves coffee first, then wine, and relishes in all things chaos.

www.SelfishMomProject.com

Made in the USA
Coppell, TX
10 January 2020

14301628R00079